9 ESSE

A S

HIP JOINT

REPLACEMENT &
SPEEDY RECOVERY

**BACK TO GETTING
PAIN-FREE – QUICKER & SAFER**

A PATIENT & PRACTITIONER'S GUIDE

VIVEK S. JAGADALE

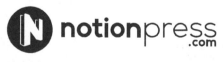

INDIA • SINGAPORE • MALAYSIA

Notion Press

Old No. 38, New No. 6
McNichols Road, Chetpet
Chennai - 600 031

First Published by Notion Press 2020
Copyright © Vivek S. Jagadale 2020
All Rights Reserved.

ISBN 978-1-64783-895-9

DISCLAIMER

Hip replacement is evolving, and demand is increasing, as is the apprehension. A recent study performed by Mayo Clinic and presented at the American Academy of Orthopedic Surgeons Annual Conference in 2014 shows that hip and knee replacement operations are among the most commonly performed operations in the USA with around one million of these procedure performed each year and another thirty to forty million joint replacement surgeries performed throughout the rest of the world every year. An estimated 4.7 million Americans have undergone total knee arthroplasty (TKA) and 2.5 million have undergone total hip arthroplasty (THA) and are living with implants as of now, with around 10% unhappy patients, families and the referring physicians due to inadequate knowledge about how to prepare and what to expect before and after this major surgery. There are so many questions in the minds of patients, families as well as consulting practitioners that remain unanswered until the date of surgery and even after. There is no good handbook or counseling book in the market that can answer all these questions from a surgeon's standpoint which would relieve their stress and help them make wise decisions. They ask: Should I get this operation? Is it safe? How long would it take before I STOP Hurting? Would I die if something goes wrong? The editors and authors of 'SUCCESSFUL Hip Joint Replacement and SPEEDY recovery' book have made every effort to provide detailed thoughtful information regarding questions about this complex and 'life-altering' surgery that is accurate and complete as of the date of publication.

To

I would like to dedicate this text to my parents who taught me that life is more than self and there is more joy in giving and sharing than taking.

To my beloved wife and son who are epitomes of love and sacrifice.

To my teachers, colleagues, trainees and patients for their constant encouragement and inspiration.

VJ

CONTENTS

Section 1

ARTHRITIS of the Hips

Section 2

SUCCESSFUL Hip Joint Replacement

Section 3

SPEEDY Recovery

PREFACE

When starting to prepare this text, we had three main objectives. The first was to write it from scratch without reference to any other passages in the hope that this would avoid the perpetuation of old errors. In doing so, we have almost certainly introduced a few new mistakes of our own which have eluded us and the reviewers. If any reader feels strongly about a point in the text, we would like them to write to us.

The second aim was to produce a book that was relevant to the patients, their families and general practitioners who get overwhelmed with the thought of major joint replacement surgery and don't know where to start, what to expect and how it would end.

Our third aim was to make it a readily available resource for everyone in this situation.

Finally, we have tried to make the text easy to read by creating a question and answer format based on the data compiled over decades from questions asked by many patients.

I firmly believe that an adequately educated patient does much better after the surgery than otherwise, and this not only makes the patient happy but also improves the overall outcomes and satisfaction.

Vivek S. Jagadale

Arkansas, USA.

ACKNOWLEDGMENT

I remain indebted to my beloved family and friends for their ongoing support, encouragement and for giving me enough time to write this book. Special thanks to my wife Akshaya; she is a wonderful life partner, mother, teacher and an even better person! Thank you!

V.J.

CONTRIBUTING AUTHORS

James R. McCoy MD

Associate Professor in Orthopedics

Central Arkansas Veterans Healthcare System, AR, USA

Ervin T. Brendl PT

Senior Therapist and Tai Chi Certified Instructor

Central Arkansas Veterans Healthcare System, AR, USA

Akshaya V. Jagadale MD

Diagnostic Radiologist

Apollo Hospitals, MS, India

Sarang S. Kasture MS, FRCS

Orthopedic Surgeon

North Bristol National Health Trust Hospital, South Wales, UK

Prashant K. Tonape MS

Arthroscopy and Joint Replacement Surgeon

Genesis Ortho, Pune, MS, India

FOREWORD

I am an eighty-nine-years-old veteran. I worked hard throughout my entire life; I was suffering from terrible left hip pain for decades, had a lot of medical issues, so no surgeon in my town was willing to perform surgery on me. I consulted and followed Dr. Jagadale's recommendations, which led to significant improvement in my overall health before the surgery, and once I got them replaced by 'Dr. Jag', my life completed changed. My pain had completely disappeared in just forty-eight hours after the muscle-sparing hip replacement surgery he did, minimal soreness remained for up to a week, and then it was like a brand new hip. Thereafter, I have felt very young and lively again with a new desire to live longer, healthier and stay busy around my grandkids. With his continuous engagement in my care and education about every step of the treatment, it was indeed a game-changer and revitalizing experience that I would look forward to witnessing it again if the need arises.

M. Federer

Hip joint replacement recipient

Bone cancer survivor

Retired navy surgeon

Section 1

❧❧

ARTHRITIS of the Hips
Pain in the Groin?

Chapter 1.1

I CAN'T WALK, CAN'T SLEEP, CAN'T EXERCISE?

Introduction

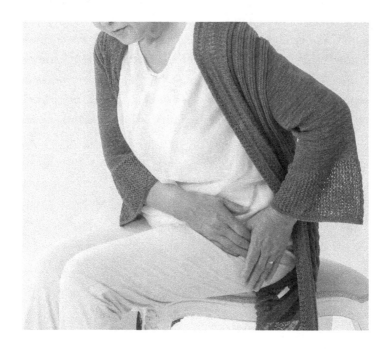

Why does my hip hurt?

In the hip, the joint is a layer of smooth cartilage on the ball of the upper end of the thighbone and another sheet within your hip socket. This cartilage functions as a cushion and allows for smooth motion of the hip. Arthritis is the wearing of this cartilage. Eventually, it wears down to the bone. Rubbing of the bone against bone causes intermittent pain (especially pain in the front of the hip joint called groin area), limping and limited walking distance.

What is arthritis (osteoarthritis)?

Osteoarthritis is a disease that affects all parts of the joint. For example, when cartilage falls apart, the bone ends start rubbing against each other. This rubbing damages your tissues and bones. The symptoms of osteoarthritis are joint pain, stiffness after you sit or lie down, and inability to move freely. Arthritis causes episodes of pain, and it may stay the same, get worse or sometimes get better over time depending on the activity level, body weight, damage inside the joint and the reason for joint damage.

Arthritis of the Hip Joint

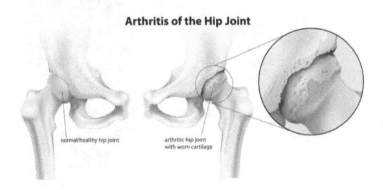

normal/healthy hip joint

arthritic hip joint
with worn cartilage

DO I HAVE BONE ON BONE ARTHRITIS?

Luxury vs. Reality

When the X-rays of the hip joint do not show any black shadow between the ball and socket, then you have bone on bone arthritis. That aching, stiff hip has shortened your quality of life. If you can't enjoy the outdoor activities you used to—like a good tennis game, a walk around the town or even playing with the grandkids—without constant pain and you have to take more than three or four over-the-counter pain pills every day to stay active and get some sleep at night, then you would benefit from a hip replacement. Hip replacement is considered as a luxury operation in patients with arthritis, and not a must-have surgery if the pain is tolerable with other treatment options are providing satisfactory pain relief. The reality is that hip pain is so unbearable at times, that the patients desperately demand surgery and once they get it in the best hands, the arthritis pain absolutely disappears. Not all patients with bone on bone arthritis hurt as bad and request a hip replacement, but when they do, it's unbearable, disabling and frustrating. The best patients are typically very old, skinny, relatively healthy and active outdoor people with strong muscles and bones. Based on the data published by the Agency for Healthcare Research and Quality, over 300,000 people undergo hip replacement surgery every year in the United States, and 90% of them do very well in expert hands. This is what the pelvis x-ray looks like in a patient with left hip joint arthritis, where bone is collapsed and the right hip joint is already replaced.

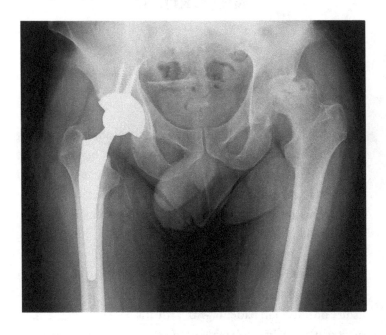

Chapter 1.3

I'M SCARED, DO I REALLY
NEED A HIP REPLACEMENT?

My family doctor says I have bone on bone disease; do I need a major surgery like hip replacement?

There are several treatment options for osteoarthritis of the hip joint depending on several factors like stage of the disease, its cause, your age, health and others. But what works for someone else may or may not be equally effective for you. Discuss with your surgeon to find what is best for you. Often a combination of things helps the most.

Treatments other than surgery include:

Medicines for pain. If your pain is mild, over-the-counter topical analgesic gels or oral pain medicines may help. These include acetaminophen (e.g., Tylenol) and nonsteroidal anti-inflammatory drugs, such as ibuprofen (e.g., Advil, Motrin) or naproxen (e.g., Aleve). But if these don't help you with satisfactory pain relief, then you may need stronger prescription medicine, (preferably non-opioid).

Low impact resistance exercise for at least forty-five minutes for three to four times a week. Water aerobics, swimming, cycling, yoga, tai-chi and similar closed chain exercises are highly recommended as they are very helpful in pain relief. They can help keep your muscles get strong, bones get tougher and your joints move well with less effort and pain.

Physical therapy to STRETCH and STRENGTHEN hip muscles. Therapy includes specific exercises that can help you stretch tightened muscles and strengthen these muscles later on so that it reduces pain and stiffness, improves mobility, joint stability and overall function.

Heat therapy vs. ice therapy in long-standing joint pain. Heating pads on the painful portion of the hip joint applied for twenty minutes every three to four hours for three to four days of increased pain may help you loosen up your joints before an activity. Ice is a good pain reliever after exercise, and heat helps in pain relief before the exercises as well as acute worsening of long-standing intermittent pain by enhancing the blood flow to the hip joint.

Walking aids help to 'OFF-LOAD' your inflamed joints. A cane (held in the opposite hand of the painful hip), a pair of crutches or a walker can help take the stress off of your hip and make it easier to get around.

Losing weight. Losing weight to bring your body mass index to thirty or less helps take some of the stress off of your joints and provides further pain relief. The easiest way to lose more than 70% of the weight is by wisely choosing healthy natural eating habits. Avoid salty, sugary, fatty, fried and processed food. Exercises, whenever possible, if done intensively for three to four days a week for thirty to forty-five minutes per session can only reduce the body weight up to 30%, and the majority of patients hurt more while doing them, so they find it more challenging.

Steroid shots for INFLAMMATION control. If you have an inflamed joint, steroid or 'rooster combs lubricant' shots in the knee can help reduce pain instantly and dramatically but the effect may be temporary. The relief usually lasts weeks to months, but if you don't have inflammation in the hip joint, then this shot won't work up to your satisfaction.

Some other things that could be considered:

Acupuncture for PAIN control. It involves inserting very tiny needles into your skin at specific places on your body to try to relieve pain. Acupuncture does not treat arthritis, but only controls pain and is not a good long-term solution. Some people find that acupuncture helps. But there is limited medical research to support the use of acupuncture for hip arthritis.

Dietary supplements available to preserve cartilage health. These are glucosamine and chondroitin, fish oil or SAM-e. Some people feel that these supplements help. But medical research does not establish that they work. Talk to your surgeon before you take these supplements.

Quitting smoking/vaping/dipping tobacco is a MUST.

Nicotine irritates the nerve endings, creates hormonal imbalances in the body, partially blocks the effect of pain medications and therefore does not give adequate pain relief. Almost all patients with tobacco in their body hurt much more, recover slower and encounter more devastating complications than the others.

Narcotics/street drugs for arthritis are a big NO-NO.

Narcotics do not control inflammation of arthritis; they numb the nerve endings in the body, create euphoria and thereby reduce the perceived pain. This pain relief is short-acting, which means after long-term use of such drugs, their effect decreases, the pain worsens, and thus medication requirement increases, dependency increases and one becomes addictive as they give a more of a sense of wellbeing which makes people partially 'forget' about the pain. That is why we do not recommend narcotics for arthritis management.

The mystery of persistent pain in the hip (referred pain).

If all these treatments do not help with the hip pain relief, then the most likely cause of your hip pain is 'neurogenic' (nerve damage from some other disease outside the hip) possibly from the lower back diseases, pelvic joint arthritis or instability, muscular weakness or neuropathy.

Section 2

❦

SUCCESSFUL Hip Joint Replacement
Am I in the Right Hands?

Chapter 2.1

AM I HEALTHY AND AM I READY?

Am I healthy and am I ready?

If you have end-stage arthritis with bone on bone disease and you are in reasonable health with no obesity, normal working heart, lungs, kidneys, blood and other major organs with no signs of infections anywhere on your body and have the desire to continue enjoying a productive life, hip replacement would be your best choice for long-standing pain relief.

Am I in the right hands?

If all medical treatment options have been tried and exhausted, then you would want to discuss surgery options with your doctor. The right surgeon is the one who has received fellowship training in total joint replacement/adult reconstructive surgeries (preferable surgical training should be done outside the country of residence for at least three months or longer) and must be at least ten years in independent orthopedic joint replacement surgery practice to expect best possible outcomes as most of them are usually at the peak of their skillsets after that time.

Am I too old, or am I too young for this type of surgery?

Either too young or too old patients might experience signs of early failure of the implant, more complications, persistent pain, infection and slower recovery as per the evidence in the scientific literature. A typical joint replacement patient is a sixty-five to eighty year old with body mass index less than thirty, free of major life-threatening health issues or immune-suppressing medications, has excellent social, mental, physical and personal health, and is independently active.

Why consider total hip arthroplasty?

Pain is interfering with routine activities and the ability to sleep.

Pain is not controlled by non-operative measures well enough that you can carry out activities of daily life comfortably.

You have tried all possible non-operative measures of pain relief, and pain is still significant.

Pain is so bad that you are willing to undergo the risks of surgery.

Goals of hip replacement

Decreased pain during normal activities (walking, sitting, sleeping)

Improved range of motion of the hip joint for better mobility, travel and daily activities

Improved hip stability (no slipping or dislocation) while reducing disability

All these changes thereby improve function, mood and social wellbeing.

Limitations

Most patients must limit certain activities (also called hip precautions) as follows:

No sitting on the ground or in the low chairs

No bending the hip beyond ninety degrees or sitting in the bucket seats

No crossing your legs

No squatting, steep climbing or forward bending

These hip precautions are critical for the first ninety days after surgery, but to be on the safe side, they should be observed throughout your lifetime.

Although surgeons strive to get your leg lengths equal, leg length is determined by the tension of the soft tissues of the hip around the new implant. Occasionally your leg might wind up longer on the operated side to ensure stability (no dislocation). If that happens, you may have to wear a shoe lift on the shorter leg.

Total hip implants only last, on average, fifteen to twenty years before they wear out and have to be revised. Revision total hip arthroplasty carries higher risks than primary (your first) total hip arthroplasty does, and it is a more technically demanding operation. Larger implants are required due to bone loss from previous surgery, and they fail much earlier than primary implants.

Some patients continue to limp even after hip replacement.

Implants in the past have been 'recalled' by the FDA for technical or medical reasons. If your implant is recalled, someone from the orthopedic service would contact you, and we would suggest what needs to be done, if anything. It is rare that a recalled implant has to be removed but can be revised if it starts giving trouble.

What is prehab? Exercises before the surgery

It is essential to be as 'fit' and 'strong' as possible before undergoing a total hip replacement. Strengthening the muscles around your hip and in your legs and arms would help to make your recovery progress faster. Good arm strength would help with using a walker and getting out of a chair during your recovery process.

Should I exercise before the surgery?

Yes. It helps to strengthen the muscles to expedite your recovery process. These simple exercises are listed below and can also be performed using ankle weights for faster gain in the function.

The exercises on the next few pages should be done as a part of your regular daily routine until at least up to six months after your surgery. If you are already doing some of these exercises, you are ahead of the game. If not, you need to begin now. You should be able to perform them in 15-twenty minutes, and we recommend that you do all of them twice a day. It is even better for you to do more as and when you can tolerate it. You can also continue with any other exercises or activities that you are doing now unless you are limited by increased pain. The instructions would tell you to count out loud. Counting out keeps you from holding your breath as you exercise.

Strengthening hip muscles:
Lying down on back – leg side-to-side movements:

Lie on your back on couch or bed and slide leg out to the side; keep toes pointed up and knee straight.

Bring the leg back to the starting point.

Repeat ten times for at least three sets two to three times a day.

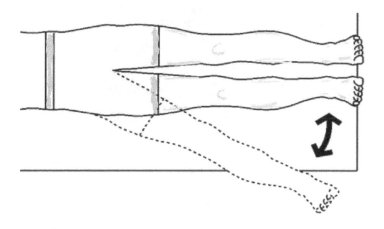

Side-lying hip - leg side-to-side movements

Lie on your side on the couch or bed, and place two pillows between your knees.

Tighten the muscle on the front of your thigh of the leg on top; you may want to bend the knee on the leg underneath.

Lift your leg six to eight inches away from the other leg (off of the pillow).

Return to starting position.

Repeat ten times for at least three sets two to three times a day.

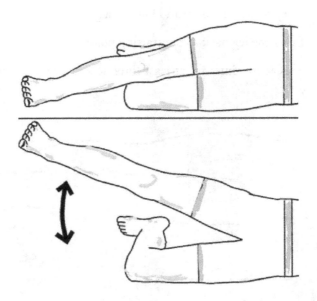

Knee straightening: long arc quads

Sit with your back against the back of the chair.

Straighten your knee as much as you can.

Slowly count to five out loud.

Relax and return to starting position.

Repeat ten times for at least three sets two to three times a day.

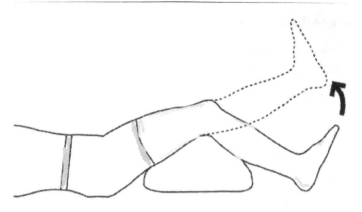

Heel slides – keeping range of motion

Lie on your back on a bed, and bend your knee and slide your heel toward your buttocks.

Slowly count to five out loud.

Relax and return to starting position.

Repeat ten times for at least three sets two to three times a day.

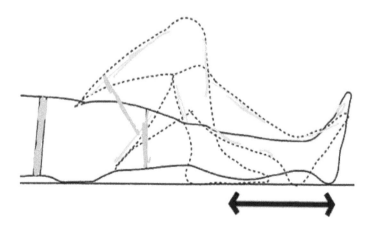

Strengthening arms

Arm exercises would help in building strength in your arms for walking with a walker or crutches.

Sit in an armchair.

Place both hands on arms rests.

Straighten your arms raising your bottom-up as much as possible.

Return to the seated position.

Repeat ten times for at least three sets two to three times a day.

Chapter 2.2

WHAT SHOULD
I ASK MY SURGEON?

Now since you have exhausted all your non-surgical treatment options, your pain is unbearable despite taking the most potent pain medications, and you have decided to pursue joint replacement surgery, it's time to find the most experienced surgeon with best hands who can deliver best surgery. Your surgeon is the ONLY key person who can explain the details of the operations, explore the benefits, risks, possible complications and recovery for your problem and alternatives, if any.

What is total hip replacement?

Total hip replacement is an operation that replaces the worn-out cartilage of the hip joint. The ball portion of the thighbone is replaced with a metal or ceramic ball on a stem that is inserted inside the femur. The socket portion is replaced with a plastic or ceramic liner that is usually fixed inside a metal shell. This fixation creates a smoothly functioning joint that does not hurt. If you have the minimally invasive approach, your recovery could be faster though in the long term, there is no difference in the outcome.

Total Hip Replacement

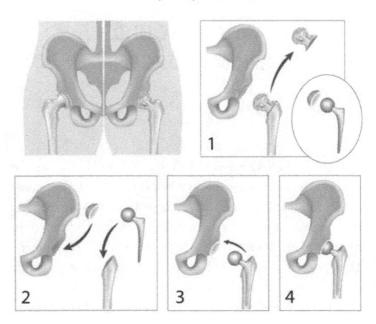

Benefits vs. risk of surgery

This is the most critical question to be asked, and then the surgeon and his team would examine you, review your X-rays, labs and other health details and discuss the best possible option available for you at that time. Hip replacement may not be ideal if your groin pain is determined to be primarily originating from your lower back or elsewhere outside your hip joint.

How long would my hip implant last, and would a second replacement be necessary?

The approximate life span of hip averages fifteen years. However, since every patient is different with a different type of arthritis, different body size, bone quality, health, muscle strength and medical issues that there is no guarantee, and some hip implants may not last that long. A revision replacement may be necessary. In general, the younger, heavier and more active patients' hips fail more quickly than the older, thinner and less active individuals. Age, weight, and activity levels are important determinants of hip arthroplasty longevity; so losing weight, eating healthier and staying fit and strong are absolutely essential.

How long does the surgery take?

Each surgeon's operative time is different. The average time in the operating room ranges from two to five hours. The actual surgical time is 1.5-2.0 hours. After the surgery, patients spend some time (about one to two hours) in the recovery room, and from there they could go home or to the nursing home depending on how fast you recover.

Would the surgery be painful?

Yes. You should expect pain at a level of 4-5 (with 0 being no pain and 10 being the worst pain you have ever felt) with your pain medication the first couple of days after surgery. This is a reasonable expectation. Every patient experiences pain differently. After surgery, the requirement of pain medication is different in different individuals, but it is lowest in those patients who are not dependent on long-term use of nicotine, narcotics, alcohol or street drugs.

What is the best type of hip replacement for me and how to find the right surgeon?

Minimally invasive direct anterior hip replacement with artificial intelligence assisted computer navigation for precision surgery is the most modern approach. This approach involves no cutting of muscles, less pain and the most promising speedy recovery in the majority of the patients in the first three to four months. Typical patients start walking with a walker on the day of the operation. Most of them go home the same evening and others in the subsequent few days depending on the complexity of the operation performed, post-surgery health and muscle strength.

The best way to find the surgeon is to ask your family practitioner, from previous patients who had the operation or find a 'joint replacement surgeon' on various search engines on the Internet. Every surgeon does this procedure slightly differently, so it would be up to the surgeon to explain his best approach, recovery and success stories.

Where would my incision be placed, and for how long?

The incision can range between three and nine inches long and would be along the front, side or back of your hip.

Would I need a walker?

Yes. Walker may be needed from a few days up to about six weeks after your surgery. We recommend you use an assistive device (rolling walker preferably), and then advance to a cane. Physical and occupational therapy services in the hospital would be able to arrange for any equipment needs, including these assistive devices, as well as bedside commodes, but regular visits to a physical therapist after discharge are not necessary as long as patients have been performing suggested exercises.

What are the significant risks with surgery?

Most surgeries go well without complications in experienced hands. However, with any type of hip replacement surgery, there are one or more risks. These include:

Dislocation of the artificial joint

Infection that requires removing the joint

Loosening of the artificial joint over time, wearing out or even implant breakage

Pneumonia

Allergic reaction to the artificial joint

Injury to nerves or blood vessels

Blood clots in the leg (deep vein thrombosis) or lungs (pulmonary embolism) which can be serious and occasionally even result in death

Mental confusion

Pressure sores

Fractures around the new prosthesis

Unequal leg lengths

Limp

Elevated levels of metal ions (metallosis) in your body which could cause adverse soft tissue and bone reactions.

Would I need blood?

With the advent of modern medicine, advanced technology and minimally invasive surgeries, the need for a blood transfusion after total joint replacement is not common but may often be required if anemia is present before the hip replacement surgery.

What would happen before my surgery?

You would meet your surgeon and anesthesiologist immediately before surgery. At that time, he or she would review all medical information to evaluate your general health. With this information, the type of anesthesia would be determined. There would be time for you to ask any questions. You would also meet your nurse, who would start the intravenous fluids along with any medications ordered to be given before the operation. Once in the operating room, you would be connected to safety monitoring devices (ECG, blood pressure cuff, pulse oximeter and other devices), You could start thinking about the sweetest experiences in your life while and the anesthesiologist is administrating the medications and shortly thereafter you would be fast asleep.

Who are anesthesiologists?

These are medical physicians that are specially trained in anesthesia. They are highly qualified and active in your care and would assist the surgical team in everything possible to keep you safe.

What types of anesthesia are available?

The anesthesia for you is specifically chosen based on your medical history.

General anesthesia, which provides loss of consciousness

Regional anesthesia, which is an injection of a local anesthetic that provides numbness and loss of pain and sensation to large areas of the body. There are medications available to you that would blur your memory.

Would I have any side effects?

Your anesthesiologist or anesthesia nurse practitioner would discuss the risks and benefits associated with the different types of anesthesia.

Nausea or vomiting may be related to the anesthesia or the type of surgical procedure you have. This is less severe now because of the advancements in anesthesia. There would be medications available to you to reduce the risk or control nausea.

Pain is another associated side effect of the surgery. The doctors and nurses can help relieve the pain through medications. No surgery is without some pain. Your pain should be tolerable, BUT DO NOT EXPECT TO BE PAIN-FREE. Please tell your caregivers about your level of pain with 1= minimal and 10=extreme.

Pain after a hip replacement

First things first, hip replacement surgery would hurt like any other major surgery. You must be prepared to experience a significant amount of discomfort in the first one to three days following surgery. First night sleep in usually rough as the pain relieving effects of medications given during surgery start fading off. Your mobility would be limited, and you would need to depend on others to help you with your regular activities of daily living. Even simple things like going to the bathroom would require assistance.

On the first day after surgery, a significant amount of surgical pain medication would be in your system. You may feel dizzy and tired. Although you had surgery on the major joint in your body, nine of ten patients would be walking on it on the same day of surgery in most of the occasions.

Be ready for the third day after your surgery. You may probably feel like you were hit by a truck. After surgery, the body sends a large number of inflammatory cells to the injured area to help with the healing process. These levels would be highest on day three. Inflammation means swelling, and swelling means pain. Talk to your surgeon about using ice and taking an anti-inflammatory medication starting on the day of surgery. But remember, typically, once patients get through day three, the swelling and pain would get better.

Walking after hip replacement surgery

Most likely, you would be up and walking with a walker on the day of or after your surgery. Take it slow and don't push yourself beyond what you can handle. Getting up and activity following surgery is vital to speeding up your recovery after a hip replacement. Try to exercise for fifteen to twenty minutes at a time three to four times a day, at least. The first day that might mean getting out of bed and to the hallway. Don't feel discouraged by this!

Moving around would speed up your recovery, increase the circulation to your legs and feet, and thereby reduce your chance of getting a blood clot. Blood clots are a serious risk following any significant surgery but can be prevented by early movement and exercise.

Getting out of bed or chair would also help to maintain and increase your muscle strength while preventing your new hip from becoming stiff. You would want to take the best advantage of that new hip movement. Don't forget that getting out of bed and walking with a walker or cane is one of the goals that you must achieve before returning home from the hospital.

General plan for surgical techniques/anesthesia/ facility/recovery

The surgeon would choose which 'brand' of an implant is right for your hip.

The representative of the company that is selling the implant would be present in the operating room to provide technical advice and support if it is needed during the surgery. This individual never touches the patient, nor does he render any clinical care whatsoever.

Anesthesia is usually general, but possibly regional, and is at the discretion of the anesthesiologist in charge of the case, upon consultation with you.

Inpatient hospitalization is typically one to three days for an uncomplicated hip replacement. Complications may prolong hospitalization.

You would have physical therapy on the same day or on post-operative day one (the day after surgery) to instruct you on how to walk with a walker. Depending on the technique the surgeon used, the quality of your bones and the initial stability of the implant, you may or may not be allowed to bear weight on your new hip.

You would go home with a bandage on the hip that would stay in place until you come back to the clinic at two weeks. You may shower (but not bathe) with the bandage on if it is waterproof and then pat it dry with a towel. If you have staples in your skin, they would be removed at your first post-operative visit.

Depending on your risk of bleeding vs. clot formation, you would be given 'sequential compression devices' to wear on the legs or medications after surgery to prevent blood clots.

If you are at higher risk for blood clots, you would be given a blood thinner starting on the day after surgery. This blood thinner is an injection that you would be taught to give yourself twice daily under the skin of your stomach.

Most patients have good results from doing their exercises at home, after instruction in the hospital. If it is determined before discharge that you need additional help from a physical therapist, this could be arranged for you.

Risk/complications

Infection: Risk is about 1%. Higher if diabetic or smoker. Infection requires removal of implants and placement of an antibiotic-impregnated spacer in the hip, plus at least six weeks of IV antibiotics. Further surgery may be necessary. A new hip cannot be implanted for at least three months, and only if lab results and clinical exams indicate that infection is cured. Absolute failure to clear the infection can result in the need to remove the antibiotic spacer and leave you without a hip joint entirely.

Measures that surgeons take to prevent infection include the following:

1. Dental clearance. A dentist must check your teeth and verify that you have no abscesses or cavities that might cause infection in your new hip. Bad teeth would have to be repaired or removed before hip replacement.

2. Skin examination. The skin of your hip, buttocks and leg must be clear and free of any scratches, bug bites or pimples. These carry bacteria and can lead to infection. If you have any skin lesions on the day of your surgery, your case would be canceled and delayed at least two weeks to allow your skin to heal up. If your planned surgical date is approaching, and you notice any skin lesions at all, call us, and we can adjust your surgery date to allow your skin to heal.

3. All sterile precautions are typically maintained throughout your hospital stay, and you are given antibiotics before the start of your surgery and for twenty-four hours afterward if you stay overnight.

Damage to nerves and vessels: very rare, but can be devastating, requiring further surgery or brace wear.

Blood clots: Blood clots are very common if no prophylaxis (preventative measures) are used. Safest are the sequential compression devices (SCDs), which wrap around your calves and periodically squeeze them gently, promoting blood flow through the veins. This, combined with a daily 325 mg Aspirin pill, has been proven to be effective (though not foolproof) in preventing blood clots in low-risk patients. If you are at increased risk for blood clots because of a medical condition or a previous blood clot, you would be given Lovenox, an injectable blood thinner. If you are already on a blood thinner, you would be instructed as to how to discontinue your usual blood thinner and use the Lovenox before and after the surgery. The use of Lovenox carries or any other blood thinner threatens for the additional risk of increased bleeding in the wound. Even with these preventative measures, a blood clot can form in your leg, and there is no adequate scientific literature that could explain this. If the clot breaks off and goes to your lungs, it can cause respiratory problems and even death. This complication is infrequent if prophylaxis (SCDs and Aspirin or blood thinner) is used. If you do get a blood clot, then prolonged use of an oral blood thinner may be necessary for up to six months.

Risks of anesthesia, including cardiac and pulmonary complications. Risks may be increased in certain patients due to specific underlying medical conditions.

Need for further surgery: A small percentage of patients get incomplete pain relief. Surgeons with fellowship training in complex joint replacement surgery can conduct a diligent search for a cause of persistent pain after total hip arthroplasty. Sometimes an infection or a technical problem is identified, such as early loosening of the prosthesis. In these cases, early revision surgery may be necessary. Often it takes a long time of watching the patient clinically before a cause for persistent pain is identified. Occasionally no cause is ever identified, and the patient must live with a certain amount of persistent pain in the hip. This problem is seen most often in patients who have lumbar spine diseases, low back surgeries with the failed back syndrome, chronic lumbar strain, and inflammation in the pelvic joints, sacroiliac joint disorders, and nerve disorders from a variety of medical issues.

Leg lengths may not feel correct, it may require a shoe lift on the opposite side.

Intraoperative fractures, breakage of the pelvis or thighbone (femur) during or immediately after the surgery is known to happen in elderly patients with osteopenia, metabolic bone diseases, less than optimal visualization in the surgical field, poor technique, trauma or fall.

Limp: Can be due to persistent of the weakness of the muscles around the hip joint from long term arthritis, occasionally from the failure of muscle repair (stitches tearing out of tissue around the bone) after surgery or leg length discrepancy.

Adverse reaction to metal ions or polyethylene (plastic) debris.

Implant failures due to wear or breakage

Joint dislocation, uncommon

Likelihood of success

Usually very good, most of the patients like the pain relief and improvement in function and health they get after surgery.

Even though the risks and complications listed above occur infrequently, they are the ones that are peculiar to the operation or of the most significant concern. The risks of surgery are similar to the risks you take every day when driving or riding in an automobile.

Any and all of these risks and complications can result in

Additional surgery

Time off work

Hospitalization

Expense to you

No guarantee – The practice of medicine and surgery is not an exact science. Although good results are anticipated, there cannot be any guarantee or warranty, express or implied, by anyone as to the results that may be obtained.

If you are using nicotine in any form, you must quit, at least three months before surgery, and preferably for the rest of your life. There is a much higher risk for poor satisfaction from outcomes, persistent pain after surgery, poor surgical site healing, early implant failure, scarring, infection and skin loss in smokers.

Checklist within thirty days of your surgery:

Pre-op appointment for medical and anesthesia clearance:

This appointment is to:

Clear you medically for the surgery by the anesthesiologist

Obtain your medical history and medications that you take at home for our hospital records

Laboratory tests, ECG, chest X-ray

Start your preoperative exercises

Home preparation for your return from the hospital:

Clean your home.

Do the laundry and put away.

Put clean linens on the bed.

Prepare meals and freeze them.

Pick up loose rugs and tack down loose carpeting.

Put a non-slip mat in the tub.

Remove electrical cords and other hazards from the hallways.

Hospital preparation

YOU MUST NOT EAT OR DRINK AFTER MIDNIGHT for an early morning surgery or preferably within the last six to eight hours before surgery as per your anesthesiologist. If you have any medication that you have been instructed to take the morning of surgery, be sure to take with a small amount of water.

Pack a bag with your personal items. Leave valuables at home.

If you wish, you may bring your clothing from home.

Types of clothing to bring

Pajamas

Shorts

Night gowns

Loose-fitting pants

Rubber-soled shoes

Don't forget:

Your notebook, storybook and a pen.

List of medications: It is not necessary to bring the actual medicines as the hospital would administer your medications from the pharmacy

Insurance cards if any

One to two days before surgery

Check your skin and toenails looking for skin lesions such as pimples, sores, abrasions, insect bites, animal bites or scratches, and ingrown toenails. **You must notify your surgeon if you see anything like this, especially if it involves the same side that is scheduled for surgery.** It puts you at an increased risk of infection. Your surgery should be re-scheduled to allow these problems to heal.

Day of surgery

In the surgical admitting area, you would be prepared for your surgery. A nurse would start your intravenous line and interview you as needed. An anesthesiologist would talk to you to gain information vital to providing anesthesia to you during your surgery. The surgeon would see you before the surgery as well. An operating room nurse would take you on a stretcher to the operating room once you are ready for surgery.

The surgeon would then perform your surgery.

Once the surgery is completed, you would be taken to the Post-Anesthesia Care Unit (PACU), where you would remain for one to three hours. During this time, a nurse would be monitoring your vital signs and your pain level. You would then be transported to your room or a similar step-down facility.

After being admitted to the hospital, you would be evaluated by a registered nurse. Your vital signs would need to be taken frequently on the first day of surgery. You would be given water first and then progress your diet as tolerated until you are ready for a regular diet.

Post-operative care in the hospital
Post-op day 1

Rise and shine on day one after surgery. Your caregivers or medical staff would assist you in getting up and out of bed to a chair or a wheelchair. If you have a drain located at the surgery site, it may be removed.

The physical therapist would assess your level of function and get you up and started walking. The role of the physical therapist is to teach you everything that would help you learn and perform the activities of daily learning after returning home. The ultimate recovery and successful outcome are based on the hard work and exercise efforts put by you at home after discharge, and the therapist only plays the role of a 'teacher/ supervisor'.

If you have an epidural catheter or a patient-controlled analgesia (PCA) pump, this would be removed in the late afternoon, and you would be switched to an oral pain medication regimen. Your coach is encouraged to be with you as much as possible. Family and friends can visit you during your hospitalization.

An incentive spirometer is a medical device that helps you perform deep breathing exercises. These exercises would help you to exercise your lungs, breathe better and improve the function of your lungs. The incentive spirometer enables you to use your lungs more effectively, deep breathing expands the lungs, aids circulation and helps prevent pneumonia.

Following are the steps to use your incentive spirometer:

Inhale normally. Relax and breathe out.

Place your lips tightly around the mouthpiece.

Make sure the device is upright.

Breathe in slowly and deeply.

Hold your breath long enough to elevate the balls (or disk) for at least three seconds.

Perform this exercise every hour while you're awake or as often as your doctor instructs.

If you were also taught coughing exercises, perform them regularly as instructed.

DVT prevention

To prevent blood clots, sequential compression devices – leg compression stockings that are placed on you after surgery and you are recommended to wear them full time except when showering for fifteen to twenty-eight days after the surgery. Compliance wear with these devices can be monitored in your best interest. In addition to this device, you would also be given other oral blood thinners (anticoagulants) as your medical condition allows.

Same-day surgery

If your surgeon feels that you are stable enough that you could go home, then this is your discharge day. Make sure you take home all the equipment that has been issued to you.

Post-op day 2

In case your stay is extended by another day, then day 2 begins with an early morning start. You are encouraged to dress in your clothes! The day usually starts with breakfast and a physical therapy session. Coaches should not hesitate to come and learn with your loved ones.

This would be the discharge day if you did not go home the day after surgery! If there are alternate plans for your discharge, your discharge planner would be assisting you in all of those arrangements.

Chapter 2.3

GOING HOME AFTER THE SURGERY?

Discharge plans

The longer you are in an acute care facility (hospital, a rehabilitation hospital or skilled nursing facility), the higher the risk of developing an infection. Early mobilization is key to a successful recovery, and being in familiar surroundings at home helps promote your activity. With those two critical aspects of your recovery in mind, the discharge plan is for you to go directly home from the hospital if at all possible.

Where would I go after discharge?

The discharge plan would be to go directly home, as mentioned earlier. Before your surgery, the surgeon usually would advise that you try to arrange to have someone stay with you for a short duration after you leave the hospital. Some patients may need to transfer to a rehab center for additional medical treatment. If you have private insurance, please review your rehab benefits before coming to the hospital. You would need to have someone drive you home on discharge day. Before leaving, your nurse would go over your detailed discharge instructions concerning medications, therapy and activities. Any special equipment (rolling walker, bedside commode etc.) would be ordered and delivered to your home.

Going to rehab or a skilled nursing facility

The decision to go to an inpatient rehabilitation facility is based on medical necessity by the recommendation of your therapist, doctor and advanced nurse practitioner.

Would I need help at home?

Yes. For the first at least two to three weeks, depending on your progress, you would need someone to assist with meal preparation, transportation, dressing, bathing and so on. Family members or friends may need to be available to help, if possible. Preparing ahead of time, before your surgery, can minimize the amount of help required.

Would I need physical therapy after I go home?

Not necessary in most of the patients who are already doing prehab. Outpatient physical therapy is not necessary for most of the hip replacement patients. There would be an exercise program given to you by the physical therapy department during your hospital stay.

How long until I can drive and return to my routine?

The ability to drive depends on the side of your surgery and what type of vehicle you drive. If the operation is on the right side, driving may be restricted for up to six weeks. 'Getting back to routine' would depend on your progress but may take up to a year or more for a patient to 'forget that he/she had a hip replacement'.

When can I return to work?

People take at least one month off from work following their joint replacement surgery. This may vary if your job is sedentary. In that case, you may return to work sooner. Please consult and discuss it with your surgeon.

How often would my doctor see me after surgery?

Ten to fourteen days after discharge, you would have a follow-up appointment with the nurse practitioner or surgeon. Routinely you would return at four weeks and three months post-op. From that point, the frequency would depend on your progress.

Do you recommend any restrictions following the surgery?

Yes. High impact activities such as running, racquetball, basketball, football, rugby, soccer, tennis, rock climbing, and mountain climbing are NOT recommended. Lifetime hip precautions (for standard total hip replacement) include:

No hip flexion greater than ninety degrees

No low chairs or overstuffed furniture

No crossing legs

Section 3

SPEEDY Recovery
When Can I Go on a Vacation?

HOW FAST CAN I GO?

Caring for yourself at home
Discomfort

After returning home, some pain is expected. You must work through a certain amount of pain to get your hip motion and thigh strength back.

Take your pain medication, preferably thirty minutes before your therapy.

Gradually wean yourself from prescription medicine to something over-the-counter.

Use ice for pain control. Do not apply ice therapy for more than twenty minutes at a time. Before and after your exercise regimen is a perfect time.

Body changes

Your appetite may be reduced. Remember to drink plenty of water and fruit juices to prevent dehydration. Your taste would return.

You may have trouble sleeping. This is common, but try not to nap too much during the day.

The energy level is decreased for the first month or two.

Pain medications tend to create constipation. To help prevent this, drink plenty of fluids, and eat fresh fruits and vegetables. Use stool softeners or laxatives if necessary. Unprocessed bran or Metamucil wafers are also helpful.

Signs of hip dislocation

Severe pain

Rotation or shortening of your leg

Inability to walk or move your leg

Signs of blood clots in the legs

Swelling in improved when the leg is elevated

Pain or tenderness in the calf (blood clots can occur in either leg)

Signs of pulmonary embolus

Sudden chest pain

Difficulty breathing

Shortness of breath

Sweating

Confusion

If this is suspected while at home, you should call 911 immediately.

Preventing infection
Precautions recommended to prevent infection

Good hand hygiene by everyone you come in contact with. The hospital staff would use alcohol-based hand foam. All visitors must clean their hands also.

Caring for your incision

Clean, sterile dressing (covering incision) needs to be left intact until your follow-up appointment with the surgeon and then would be removed.

White dressing (covering drain wound) needs to be kept clean and dry until there is no drainage, and the drain hole has scabbed over. Then the patient may remove white dressing and shower.

Avoid massaging, scratching, or oiling, touching or allowing others to reach your incision until the skin sutures or staples are off, and your incision has healed. ONLY FRESHLY WASHED HANDS OR HEALTH CARE PROVIDERS WEARING GLOVES TOUCH INCISIONS. Showering may be allowed if the surgical site dressing is waterproof or is completely covered with plastic, but sinking the surgical site in a tub or pool is not recommended.

Lifetime infection prevention

Although the risks are low for long-term infections after hip replacement surgery, it is essential to realize that the threat remains.

A prosthetic joint could attract the bacteria from an infection located in another part of your body. Be sure to see your family practitioner for any illness and finish any antibiotics if prescribed.

It is recommended you take an antibiotic before any invasive procedure, which would include dental cleaning and other invasive dental procedures as well as any invasive surgery or procedures such as a colonoscopy or instrumentation of your urinary tract.

Notify your surgeon immediately for any of these changes:
Signs of infection

Increased redness or swelling at the surgical site

Change in color, odor or amount of drainage

Increased pain in the hip

Fever is expected during the first five to seven days after a major surgery as your body is recovering. After that time, notify your physician.

Continue to use your incentive spirometer, and coughing and deep breathing techniques as this would decrease your risk of pneumonia.

Chapter 3.2

EXERCISE, EXERCISE, EXERCISE?

Therapist as an exercise teacher
Activity guidelines

Exercise is vital to help you obtain the best possible results from your hip surgery. You should begin doing exercises with the therapist on the first day after your operation. The next few pages contain some guidelines for your post-operative activity and exercise program. Your therapist would personalize these for you if necessary.

Total hip replacement post-surgery exercise plan
Weeks 2-4 (for standard total hip replacement)

During the weeks one and two of your recovery, your goals are:

Continue walking with a walker or two crutches unless otherwise instructed.

Walk at least two hundred to four hundred feet with a walker or crutches daily.

Walk up and down curbs and ramps.

Actively bend your hip up to sixty degrees.

Straighten your hip completely.

Independently sponge bathe or shower and dress, maintain hip precautions.

Gradually resume light household tasks.

Twice a day, do the home exercises program given to you.

Total hip replacement post-surgery exercise plan Weeks 4–6 (standard total hip replacement)

By this time, you would be feeling confident and comfortable with your new hip, but you are still recovering, and maximum benefit is the goal. Continuing to be goal-oriented and committed to your home exercise program is essential.

Your goals for this period are:

Achieve all of the goals listed from weeks 1-2 if not yet accomplished.

Use an assistive device such as walker or crutches for the first six weeks after surgery – you would be touch down weight bearing (TDWB), meaning operative leg may touch the floor for balance, but no weight is to be applied through it.

Walk a quarter to half a mile daily.

Actively bend hip.

Continue with the home exercise program twice a day.

Total hip replacement post-op exercise plan Weeks 6-12 (for standard total hip replacement)

During weeks 6-12, you should be able to resume regular activity and perhaps even add some that you could not do before surgery.

Your goals for this period are:

Achieve all prior goals if not yet accomplished.

Walk with no cane or crutch and without a limp.

Climb and descend stairs in a typical fashion (foot over the foot).

Walk a half to a full mile daily.

Resume all activities including dancing, bowling and golf (closer to week 12).

For minimally invasive surgery – direct anterior hip replacement*

Weeks 1-2

Full weight-bearing as tolerated

Walker or crutches (mostly just for balance)

Week 2-12

Progress to cane in opposite hand (for balance only)

No assistive device if you are stable walking

Have good strength and balance.

- You may resume essentially normal activities as tolerated and drive once off all narcotic medications.

- Usually, no hip activity precautions or physical therapy are needed.

- You would need to follow all infection, and blood clot prevention strategies described earlier in the standard total hip protocol.

Chapter 3.3

RECOVERY AND RETURN TO RECREATION

Loving thy hip, wife, and life

Usually, after five to seven days after the surgery, most of the patients stop taking pain medications on a routine basis, are relatively active with minimal pain, and start enjoying their return to activities of daily living.

How long would I be incapacitated?

You would begin walking the very same day or next day after hip replacement. If you have an MIS (minimally invasive surgery) direct anterior option, your activity can be expedited. Usually, you would start out using a walker or two crutches, which may be needed for 2-12 weeks depending upon your particular situation.

What physical/sport activities may I participate in after my recovery?

You may participate in walking, dancing, golf, hiking, swimming, bowling and gardening upon clearance from your surgeon. These activities are encouraged to help you return to a relatively pain-free, functional lifestyle.

Lifetime hip precautions
Hip precautions while standing or walking

Don't cross your legs at any time!

Don't let the knee of your affected leg go past your belly button.

Don't extend your affected leg back behind you or out to the side.

Don't turn the foot of your operated leg inward (pigeon towed).

Don't stoop or squat.

Don't turn your shoulders or twist at the waist toward your affected leg while keeping your foot still. Lift your foot on the affected leg and turn your whole body in the direction of your affected limb. The most common mistake patients make twisting their bodies while keeping one leg still.

When turning, take small steps in the direction you want to turn mainly using your 'good' leg. Don't reach for objects by turning your shoulders without also turning your pelvis.

Don't step up on a stair/surface where your knee would be higher than your hips.

Don't kneel on the knee of the unaffected leg (good leg). Do kneel on the knee of the affected limb.

If you had an anterior approach – do not allow the knee of the affected leg to go behind your hip when walking.

Hip precautions while sitting

Don't cross your legs at any time!

Don't sit in a way that your hips are at the same level or lower than your knees.

Don't lean forward when you are moving to sit down or rock forward when standing up from a sitting position.

Don't lean forward while you are sitting down, as in reaching for something.

Don't sit in recliners. Recliners are hard to stand up from without leaning or rocking your body forward.

Add a firm pillow to your seat to keep your hips higher than your knees.

Sit in chairs that have arms. As you sit down or stand up, use the chair's arms for support and to control your movement. This type of chair takes the pressure off of your legs and hips. It can also prevent you from wanting to lean forward for balance or rock forward to stand up.

Don't lean forward to pick things up from the floor.

Do get up and go for a short walk at least once every hour.

Hip precautions while lying down

Don't cross your legs at any time!

Don't pull your knees towards your chest.

Don't let the foot of your operated leg turn inward.

Don't lie on the side; you had your hip replacement. If you sleep on your unaffected side, keep a pillow between your legs to keep them from crossing. Also, be sure your foot is rested on the pillow so that the toes don't dangle and turn inward.

Don't lean forward when resting in bed, such as adjusting blankets or pillows.

Do sleep on your back with a wide pillow between your legs. Many people ask if they can sleep on their stomachs after hip replacement. The problem with sleeping on your stomach is that it causes your feet to turn too far out or in. When your feet turn too far out or in, the ball of your hip joint is at risk for popping out of the joint socket. After the ligaments and muscles in your hip have had a chance to heal for several months, ask your surgeon if it is OK for you to sleep on your stomach.

Do not bend your hip beyond ninety degrees. Don't pull knees to your chest.

Do not turn your foot inward.

Do not cross your legs.

Hip precautions during activities of daily living

Restrictions on your movement affect your daily activities and how you do them.

Use pain as a guide to what you can and cannot do.

Use ice to reduce pain and swelling.

Place a wedge or two pillows between your knees when sleeping on your non-operative side. The pillows or a wedge would prevent you from crossing your legs in your sleep. You should sleep with the pillow between your legs for six weeks.

Use a raised toilet seat. A raised toilet seat can prevent you from rocking your body forward when standing up. Getting up from a low toilet seat is a common cause of hip dislocation.

Add temporary handrails or grab bars in areas where you need support, such as near the toilet, shower or tub.

Don't get down into the bathtub. A unique bench can be used to straddle the side of the tub that you can sit on while you bathe. Adjust the seat, so your hips are higher than your knees when sitting.

Use reaching aids to bathe. You should not bend over or forward to wash.

Use an adjustable shower stool to prevent falls. Be sure to adjust the height, so your hips are higher than your knees when sitting.

Have someone help put your socks and shoes on. Bending over to do it yourself puts your hip joint in a position that could easily cause it to dislocate.

Use a reaching aid to help with dressing. Don't bend down to pull up your pants or tie your shoes.

Don't reach down to pick something up while sitting.

Don't lift more than thirty pounds. Anything you lift adds weight that your new hip replacement must support.

Don't drive for at least six to eight weeks following hip surgery. When riding as a passenger, you may need to add a pillow in the seat to get your hips higher than your knees. Place a plastic bag on the seat. This plastic helps you to slide out of the car quickly without having to lean or rock forward.

Do limit stair climbing. When climbing up the stairs, the 'good' leg should step first and then bring the affected leg up to the same step. Then bring up your crutches or cane. When going down the stairs, first put your crutches or cane on the lower step, then put your affected leg down to the next step, and finally, step down to the same step with your 'good' leg.

Accomplishing activities of daily living
Standing up from a chair

Do NOT pull up on the walker to stand. Sit in a chair with armrests when possible. Initially, keep operative leg forward when standing or sitting.

Scoot to the front edge of the chair.

Push up with both hands on the armrests.

If sitting in a chair without armrests, place one hand on the walker while pushing off the side of the chair with the other.

Balance yourself before grabbing the walker.

Walking with a walker

Move the walker forward.

With all four legs of walker firmly on the ground stable, step forward with the operative leg and place the foot in the middle of the walker area; DO NOT move it past the front feet of the walker.

Put some of the weight on your arms and step forward with the non-operated leg.

Repeat.

NOTE: Take small steps and be sure that all four legs/wheels of the walker are firmly on the ground before stepping.

Lying in bed

You should keep your operated knee as straight as possible while you are lying in bed.

Lie on your back. Put a small pillow under your ankle and lower leg, but NOT UNDER YOUR KNEE; keep your knee as straight as possible.

If you are going to lie on your side, you may be more comfortable with a pillow between your knees, but again, keep your operated knee as straight as possible.

Getting in and out of bed
Getting in bed

Back up to the edge of the bed until you feel it on the back of your legs.

You need to be halfway between the foot and the head of the bed.

Reaching back with both hands, sit on the edge of the bed and then scoot back toward the center of the mattress (silk pajamas, satin sheets, or sitting on a plastic bag may make it easier).

Move your walker out of the way but keep it in reach.

Lift your leg into the bed while scooting around, or you may need someone to assist you if this is your operated leg, but if no one else is available, you may use a leg lifter, cane, rolled bed sheet or belt to assist you in getting this leg into the bed.

Lift your other leg as you keep scooting.

Continue scooting your hips into the center of the bed.

CAUTION: DO NOT ever cross your legs to assist with getting the operated leg in and out of bed.

Getting out of bed

Scoot your hips to the side of the bed.

Sit up while lowering your outside leg to the floor. If necessary, use a leg lifter, cane, rolled bed sheet or belt to assist you.

Once both feet are on the floor, scoot your hips to the edge of the bed.

Place your operated leg slightly in front of the non-operated leg.

Position the walker in front of yourself.

Use both hands to push off the surface of the bed. If the mattress is too low, place one hand in the center of the walker while pushing off the bed with the other hand.

Balance yourself before grabbing the walker.

Sitting and rising from the toilet
Sitting down on the toilet

Take small steps to turn until your back is to the toilet. Do NOT pivot.

Back up to the toilet until you feel it touch the back of your leg.

Slide your operated leg out in front of you.

If you are using a commode with armrests, reach back for both armrests and lower yourself onto the toilet.

Getting up from the toilet:

If using a commode with armrests, use the armrests to push up with both hands; make sure your operated leg is slightly in front of the other leg when coming to standing.

Balance yourself before grabbing the walker.

Getting into the car

Push the car seat back; recline the seat if possible but return it to the upright position for traveling.

Place a plastic trash bag in the seat of the car to help you slide and turn frontward.

Back up to the vehicle until you feel it touch the back of your knees.

Reach back for the car seat and lower yourself down, keep your operated leg straight out in front of you and bend your head so that you don't hit it on the doorframe.

Turn frontward, while leaning back as you lift the operated leg into the car.

Putting on pants and underwear:

Sit down.

Put your operated leg in first, then put your non-operated leg.

Use a dressing stick or a reacher to guide the waistband over your foot.

Pull your pants up over your knees, so that it is within reach.

Stand with the walker placed in front of you to pull your pants up the rest of the way.

Taking off pants and underwear:

Back up to the chair or bed where you would be undressing.

Unfasten your pants and let them drop to the floor.

Push your underwear down to your knees.

Lower yourself down, keeping your operated leg out straight.

Take your non-operated leg out first and then the operated leg.

Putting on socks
To use a sock aid:

Sit down.

Slide the sock onto the sock aid.

Hold the cord and drop the sock aid in front of your foot; it is easier to do this if your knee is bent as much as possible.

Slip your foot into the sock aid.

Straighten your knee, point your toe and pull the sock on.

Keep pulling until the sock aid pulls out of the socks.

Note: You must not cross your legs when putting on your socks.

Putting on shoes

1. Use your reacher, dressing stick or long-handled shoehorn to slide your shoe in front of your foot; bend your knee backward as much as possible when doing this.

NOTE: Wear sturdy slip-on shoes or shoes with Velcro closures or elastic shoelaces. Do NOT wear high-heeled shoes without backs. Tennis shoes can be challenging to put on. Loafer style shoes are easier to put on.

Tips for household chores:
Saving energy and protecting your joints
When working in the kitchen:

Do NOT get down on your knees to scrub floors; instead, use a mop and long-handled brushes.

Plan ahead! Gather all of your cooking supplies at one time, then, sit to prepare your meal.

Place frequently used cooking supplies and utensils where they can be reached without too much bending or stretching (usually between waist and shoulder height).

To provide better working height, use a sturdy high stool, or put cushions on your chair when preparing meals.

When cleaning the bathroom:

Do NOT get down on your knees to scrub the bathtub.

Use a mop or other long-handled brushes.

Safety and avoiding falls Follow these safety precautions for all areas of your home
Before your surgery:

Pick up throw rugs and tack down loose carpeting.

Cover slippery surfaces with carpet that are firmly anchored to the floor or have non-skid backs.

Provide good lighting throughout the house and if needed, install nightlights in the bathrooms, bedrooms and hallways.

After your surgery and in general:

Be aware of all floor hazards such as pets, small objects or uneven surfaces.

Keep extension cords out of pathways.

Sit in chairs with armrests as this would make it easier for you to get up.

Rise slowly from either a sitting or lying position so as not to get light-headed.

Do not lift heavy objects for the first three months, and then only with your surgeon's permission.

Let friends and family know to allow you extra time to get to the phone.

Stop and think, use good judgment – do not be in a hurry.

Life-long exercise

Whether you have reached all the recommended goals in three months or not, all joint patients need to have a regular exercise program to maintain their fitness and the health of the muscles around their joints.

With both your orthopedic and family practitioner's permission, you should be on a regular exercise program three to four times per week lasting twenty to thirty minutes.

Impact activities, such as running and singles tennis, may put too much load on the joint and are not recommended. High-risk activities such as downhill skiing are discouraged because of the risk of fractures around the prosthesis.

What to do for exercise:

Low-impact exercise classes

Home program as outlined in this notebook.

Regular one to three-mile walks

Home treadmill walking

Regular exercise at a fitness center

Arthritis aquatic classes

What NOT to do for exercise?

Do not run or engage in high impact activities (jogging, racquet sports, basketball, football, rugby, soccer, singles tennis, rock climbing, mountain biking, etc.).

Do not participate in high-risk activities such as downhill skiing.

When can I start making love after hip replacement?

Yes, it is a question every patient has but often hesitates to ask. Check with your surgeon, but it is usually safe to resume sexual activity six weeks to eight weeks following a standard hip replacement. Remember, as with all businesses, to listen to your body! You should not attempt to do more than you feel capable of and to stop or slow down if you notice increased pain. During the act, preferably keep the legs closer to the body to minimize the risk of hip dislocation and other complications.

Do's and don'ts after a hip replacement

The do's and don'ts might be different depending on what type of surgical technique your doctor used. Your doctor and your physical therapist can give you a specific list to remember. These precautions are standard to prevent your new hip from dislocating and to help with a quick and thorough recovery.

How long until you feel 'normal' after a hip replacement?

Hip replacement is an excellent option to improve your health and quality of life, but it would take time before you are functional. The literature reports that 90% of patients who undergo a hip replacement stated the procedure was successful. They reported complete relief from hip pain and were able to be more active and connect with their loved ones following the surgery.

These results are very encouraging, but it is not an overnight cure. You can expect to wait for 10-12 weeks before you can return to all your favorite activities. At some point, you may feel like your recovery is taking too long. It's important to remind yourself that feeling limited and frustrated with physical ability are a normal part of the healing process. It may take up to a year or more before you 'forget' that you had a hip replacement.

Take a break and slow down a little bit rather than pushing yourself. Do something you can enjoy. Get help if needed, think about how far you have already come, then get back up, keep moving and eating healthy. 10-12 weeks would feel like a very long time, but once you are enjoying a pain-free stroll, that time would be just a memory.

So, read & follow this guide, relax, re-organize and reap the benefits of your brand new hip joint and it will make you 'feel' younger, healthier and happier again to enjoy the life you always wanted.

Wishing You a Bon Voyage &

Speedy Recovery (English)

जल्द स्वस्थ (Hindi)

विनाविलंब पुनर्प्राप्ती (Marathi)

જલ્દી સાજુ થવું (Gujarati)

Reprise rapide (French)

Schnelle Erholung (German)

Recuperación rápida (Spanish)

Recuperatis (Latin)

BLURB

PAIN from arthritis can be troubling, disruptive and depressive. Hip joint replacement for arthritis of a hip joint is like a heart transplant for a damaged heart. It is evolving, and demand is increasing, as is the apprehension. This book gives a precise approach, guidance and education on how to overcome fear, what to expect, and how to cope up with the surgery faster and safer. This book is extremely valuable for a patient or a family member or a doctor who is trying to help a patient with arthritis. Most of the pain-controlling options are temporary and unsatisfactory. Hip joint replacement is the best long-term solution to end-stage arthritis. There are so many questions in the minds of patients, families as well as consulting practitioners that remain unanswered until the surgery is scheduled and occasionally even after leading to less than desired outcomes. There is no good single resource or handbook in the market that can answer all these questions from a real surgeon's standpoint which will help alleviate the stress and help patients and their families make wise, informed decisions. They ask: I am scared of operations but my pain is terrible, should I get this operation? Is it safe? How long will it take before I STOP Hurting? Will I die if something goes wrong? The editors and authors of '9 Most Essential Answers of SUCCESSFUL Hip Joint Replacement & SPEEDY recovery' book have made every effort to provide detailed, thoughtful information regarding questions about this complex and 'life-altering' surgery that is accurate and complete as of the date of publication.

I firmly believe that an adequately educated patient and family do much better with the treatment provided in the best possible way than otherwise. It not only makes the patient happy but also improves their outlook, recovery speed, overall outcomes and satisfaction.

NOTES